T0336270

Cambridge Elements ≡

Elements in Emergency Neurosurgery
edited by
Nihal Gurusinghe
Lancashire Teaching Hospital NHS Trust
Peter Hutchinson
University of Cambridge, Society of British Neurological Surgeons and Royal College of Surgeons of England
Ioannis Fouyas
Royal College of Surgeons of Edinburgh
Naomi Slator
North Bristol NHS Trust
Ian Kamaly-Asl
Royal Manchester Children's Hospital
Peter Whitfield
University Hospitals Plymouth NHS Trust

MILD TRAUMATIC BRAIN INJURY INCLUDING CONCUSSION

Thomas D. Parker
Imperial College London

Colette Griffin
St George's Hospital NHS Trust

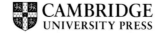

CAMBRIDGE
UNIVERSITY PRESS

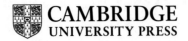

Shaftesbury Road, Cambridge CB2 8EA, United Kingdom

One Liberty Plaza, 20th Floor, New York, NY 10006, USA

477 Williamstown Road, Port Melbourne, VIC 3207, Australia

314–321, 3rd Floor, Plot 3, Splendor Forum, Jasola District Centre, New Delhi – 110025, India

103 Penang Road, #05–06/07, Visioncrest Commercial, Singapore 238467

Cambridge University Press is part of Cambridge University Press & Assessment, a department of the University of Cambridge.

We share the University's mission to contribute to society through the pursuit of education, learning and research at the highest international levels of excellence.

www.cambridge.org
Information on this title: www.cambridge.org/9781009476058

DOI: 10.1017/9781009380089

First published 2023

A catalogue record for this publication is available from the British Library

ISBN 978-1-009-47605-8 Hardback
ISBN 978-1-009-38009-6 Paperback
ISSN 2755-0656 (online)
ISSN 2755-0648 (print)

Cambridge University Press & Assessment has no responsibility for the persistence or accuracy of URLs for external or third-party internet websites referred to in this publication and does not guarantee that any content on such websites is, or will remain, accurate or appropriate.

Mild Traumatic Brain Injury including Concussion

Elements in Emergency Neurosurgery

DOI: 10.1017/9781009380089
First published online: December 2023

Thomas D. Parker
Imperial College London

Colette Griffin
St George's Hospital NHS Trust

Author for correspondence: Thomas D. Parker, t.parker@imperial.ac.uk

Abstract: Most traumatic brain injury (TBI) cases are considered mild. Precise definitions vary, but typically, loss of consciousness and post-traumatic amnesia duration is brief (e.g. <30 minutes and <24 hours, respectively), and standard imaging is normal. Prognosis in mild TBI is generally good, but disabling persistent symptoms such as headache, dizziness, and affective and cognitive issues are common. A focussed assessment tailored to each individual symptom is crucial for management. Advanced MRI and blood-based biomarkers of mild TBI are emerging and are likely to play an increasingly important role in the assessment of patients following a head injury.

Keywords: head injury, mild traumatic brain injury, concussion, imaging, management

ISBNs: 9781009476058 (HB), 9781009380096 (PB), 9781009380089 (OC)
ISSNs: 2755-0656 (online), 2755-0648 (print)

Contents

Epidemiology, Definitions, and Classification of Mild TBI

Approximately 1.4 million patients attend accident and emergency with head injury in England and Wales (1). Data from the Trauma Audit and Research Network has revealed that the vast majority of patients with a traumatic brain injury (TBI) are defined as 'mild' (2). Definitions of what constitutes a mild TBI vary. The criteria proposed by the World Health Organization Collaborating Center Task Force on Mild TBI considers an individual to have experienced a mild TBI after a head injury if they have a documented Glasgow Coma Scale (GCS) score of 13–15 at presentation to hospital and/or a loss of consciousness <30 minutes duration and/or post-traumatic amnesia <24 hours (3). The Mayo Clinic classification system of TBI (Table 1, (4) has a similar approach, but also incorporates information from imaging findings. According to the Mayo Clinic classification, a patient is said to have experienced a mild (probable) TBI if they have at least one of the following: a loss of consciousness of less than 30 minutes duration; post-traumatic amnesia of less than 24 hours; and normal standard imaging (excluding a depressed, basilar, or linear skull fracture with intact dura). An absence of loss of consciousness or post-traumatic amnesia would place the patient in the symptomatic (possible) category. However, mild (probable) and symptomatic (possible) are often jointly referred to as 'mild TBI' (5). Death, loss of consciousness of greater than 30 minutes, post-traumatic amnesia of greater than 24 hours, a documented GCS score of <13 in the first 24 hours, or any of the imaging abnormalities detailed in Table 1 would place the patient in the moderate–severe (definite) category. The rationale for excluding individuals with abnormal imaging findings from the 'mild TBI' group is supported by work that revealed that evidence of contusion, subarachnoid heamorrhage, and/or subdural heamatoma on CT scanning predicted incomplete recovery in patients with mild TBI classified on GCS scores alone (GCS score of 13–15) (6).

The term mild TBI is often used interchangeably with the term concussion (5). A precise definition of concussion has not been established, but it is often considered to be a syndrome, including a wide range of symptoms such as headache, dizziness, fatigue, irritability, reduced concentration, sleep disturbance, memory impairment, anxiety, depression, photophobia, and phonophobia. It is not uncommon for a patient with such a constellation of symptoms to be diagnosed with a concussion and given simple reassurance, which can be problematic. Firstly, although prognosis in mild TBI is generally good with most

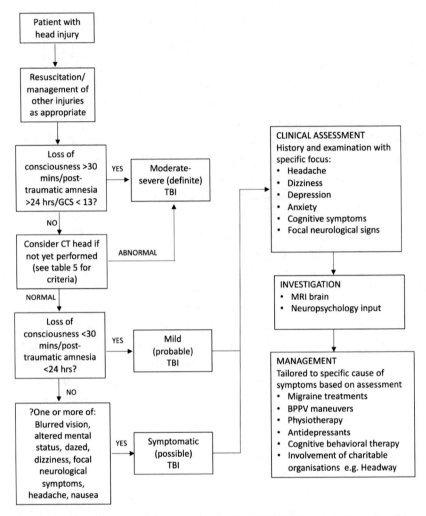

Figure 1 Algorithm providing overview of mild TBI diagnosis, investigation, and management.

patients recovering in the first three months, many report on-going symptoms persisting beyond six months (7), which challenges the concept that the natural history of concussion is one of relatively quick and benign recovery. It should be noted that many argue that the term 'mild' in mild TBI is also somewhat of misnomer in this context as well and does not capture the significant physical, cognitive, and psychosocial morbidity that can occur (8). Secondly, this approach often precludes more detailed clinical assessment of individual symptoms, which in turn limits the ability to address individual symptoms by instituting tailored

Table 1 Mayo Clinic classification system of TBI (4)

Mayo Clinic classification of TBI – category	Criteria
Moderate–severe (definite)	One or more of the following: • Death due to this TBI • Loss of consciousness >30 minutes • Post-traumatic anterograde amnesia >24 hours • Worst GCS in first 24 hours <13 (unless invalidated by other factors such as intoxication, sedation, and systemic shock) • Evidence of one of the following: intra-cerebral haematoma, subdural haematoma, epidural haematoma, cerebral contusion, haemorrhagic contusion, penetration of dura, subarachnoid haemorrhage, or brainstem injury
Mild (probable)	Does not fulfil any criterion of moderate–severe (definite) TBI plus one of the following: • Loss of consciousness <30 minutes • Post-traumatic anterograde amnesia <24 hours • Depressed, basilar, or linear skull fracture (dura intact)
Symptomatic (possible)	Does not fulfil any criterion of moderate–severe (definite) TBI *or* mild (probable) plus one or more of the following: • Blurred vision • Confusion (mental state changes) • Daze • Dizziness • Focal neurological symptoms • Headache • Nausea

strategies (see Figure 1 for overview). A prime example being dizziness, which may be a result of brain injury, vestibular migraine, or peripheral vestibular dysfunction, all of which necessitate a tailored diagnostic and management approach (5).

Clinical Presentations and Management of Mild TBI

Loss of Consciousness

Establishing whether a patient has lost consciousness following a head injury is a key component of TBI classification and assessment. However, precisely defining loss of consciousness can be challenging, especially in retrospect. Collateral information from an eyewitness, paramedics, CCTV, or even a patient's personal electronic device can be helpful. It is also important to interpret a history of loss of consciousness in the context of other potential confounds, such as drugs (illicit or prescribed, including anaesthesia) and hypovolaemia (e.g. from trauma-related blood loss). It is also important to consider whether any loss of consciousness was the product of a head injury or the root cause. Seizures and cardiac causes of syncope are a common cause of head injury and the absence of appropriate investigation and management places the patient at risk of further events and potential further injury and death.

Post-traumatic Amnesia

Post-traumatic amnesia is usually defined as the period between a head injury and the return of normal episodic memory function (9). However, other features are often prominent and include disorientation, behavioural disturbance, inattention, slowed processing speed, and executive dysfunction. Epidemiology studies have shown that post-traumatic amnesia is a key prognostic indicator following a TBI and is much more informative than other variables such as consciousness level (10). Post-traumatic amnesia often goes unrecognised and it can be a difficult diagnosis to make, especially in retrospect. Detailed information from a collateral source is vital and it is important to take into account potential confounders such as pre-existing cognitive impairment and other causes of delirium, such as drugs, infection, and metabolic abnormalities. Although not without their limitations, validated tools such as the Westmead PTA scale, which includes a combination of orientation questions and delayed recall questions, can be administered relatively quickly in an acute setting and are useful for accurately identifying post-traumatic amnesia. Psychotropic medications such as benzodiazepines and anti-psychotics should be avoided and management should focus on providing a calm, reassuring environment, whilst providing regular orientating and familiarising information (11).

Headache

Headache is a common issue following mild TBI, with prospective studies estimating 91% of patients reporting new or worsening headaches compared to pre-injury at some point in the 12 months post-injury, with migraine being the most common cause (12). The site, onset, character, associated symptoms, time course, exacerbating and relieving factors, as well as the severity of the headache, are all important components of the history that enable accurate phenotype characterisation. A positive diagnosis of migraine is particularly helpful as it allows specific management. Diagnostic criteria for migraine are highlighted in Table 2. Red flags for causes of secondary headache (which may or may not be related to the original head injury) such as thunderclap presentation, focal neurological symptoms/signs, optic disc swelling, pulsatile tinnitus, fever, and neck stiffness are important to identify.

Management of migraine is divided into acute and chronic treatments. A combination of a triptan (e.g. sumatriptan, which can be given orally or subcutaneously, or rizatriptan, which is available in preparations that dissolve in the mouth) with one simple analgesic agent (e.g. a non-steroidal anti-inflammatory drug or paracetamol) and a antiemetic/prokinetic (e.g domperidone, metoclopramide, or prochlorperazine) is favoured for acute management (14). Very frequent use of acute migraine treatments runs the risk of medication-overuse headache and should be avoided. In particular, it is vital to avoid opioid medications as they also increase the risk of medication-overuse headache, are addictive, and have harmful side effects that may exacerbate other symptoms related to the mild TBI, such as drowsiness, dizziness, constipation, and cognitive issues. For chronic migraine (defined as headaches on >15 days a month, for over 3 months, and with migrainous headaches on >8 days a month), migraine-prophylactic agents are indicated (14). There are a wide

Table 2 *The International Classification of Headache Disorders*, 3rd edition, crtieria for migraine without aura (13)

Diagnostic criteria for migraine without aura

A   At least five attacks fulfilling criteria B–D
B   Headache attacks lasting 4–72 hours (untreated or unsuccessfully treated)
C   Headache has at least two of the following four characteristics:
   1. Unilateral location
   2. Pulsating quality
   3. Moderate or severe pain intensity
   4. Aggravation by or causing avoidance of routine physical activity (e.g. walking or climbing stairs)
D   During headache at least one of the following:
   1. Nausea and/or vomiting
   2. Photophobia and phonophobia
E   Not better accounted for by another diagnosis

Table 3 Migraine prophylactic agents

Drug	Mechanism of action	Important side effects
Propranolol	Beta-blocker	Bradycardia, hypotension, erectile dysfunction, bronchospasm (important to avoided in COPD/asthma)
Topiramate	Anti-epileptic	Weight loss, cognitive slowing, and renal stones
Candesartan	Angiotensin II receptor blocker	Hypotension
Amitriptyline	Tri-cyclic antidepressant	Sedating (although may be helpful in individuals with sleep difficulties), can lower seizure threshold
Nortriptyline	Tri-cyclic antidepressant	As per amitriptyline, but less sedating
Duloxetine	Serotonin and norepinephrine reuptake inhibitor	Constipation, diarrhoea, weight gain, hypertension
Pizotifen	Serotonin antagonist	Drowsiness, weight gain, dry mouth, urinary retention

range of well-established medications that are potentially useful, and some commonly prescribed examples are detailed in Table 3. More recently, treatments such as botulinum toxin and calcitonin gene-related peptide monoclonal antibodies have also been shown to be highly effective in migraine prevention, particularly in patients who have not responded to standard prophylactic agents, and are largely prescribed by headache specialists. Many also advocate the use of certain daily over-the-counter nutritional supplements such as magnesium, riboflavin, and coenzyme Q10, which can be used in combination with standard prescribed therapies.

Dizziness

Dizziness is a common symptom following mild TBI and can be challenging to disentangle but is highly treatable. There is a broad differential and patients often find it difficult to describe their symptoms, which at times limits the usefulness of focussing on the precise nature of the dizziness (e.g. 'true rotational vertigo' compared to 'light-headedness'). The tempo of the symptoms and associated symptoms are often the most important part of the history.

One of the most common causes of dizziness/vertigo post head injury is benign paroxysmal positional vertigo (BPPV), which is felt to occur due to mechanical displacement of calcium carbonate 'crystals' or otoconia during a head injury. Recurrent episodes of dizziness/vertigo that last seconds at time in specific positions are highly suggestive of BPPV. Posterior canal BPPV is the most common form, which typically manifests as delayed onset up beating, torsional, fatigueable nystagmus during Dix–Hallpike testing. Multi-canal BPPV is more common in the context of trauma so it is important to perform Dix–Hallpike testing bilaterally. A supine log roll is recommended to screen for horizontal canal BPPV (15). There are a range of positional manoeuvres that can be used to treat BPPV, such as the Epley or Semont; they can be performed immediately at the point of diagnosis and are highly effective (16). Referral to vestibular physiotherapy may also be helpful, especially if symptoms are prolonged and resistant to simple manoeuvres.

Vestibular migraine is another highly common cause of vertigo post head injury, which typically presents as prolonged episodes of dizziness with associated headache and migrainous features (Table 2) and can be treated with migraine prophylatics (Table 3).

Although debilitating, most cases of dizziness are benign. However, it is vital to consider posterior circulation stroke, especially in patients presenting with acute onset persistent dizziness, which may be secondary to vertebral artery dissection in the context of a recent head injury, particularly if examination findings suggestive of cerebellar or brainstem dysfunction are present. Investigations of choice are MRI brain with DWI sequences, as well as vessel imaging (CT angiogram or MR angiogram). A plain CT head has limited sensitivity and is not sufficient to exclude a posterior circulation stroke.

Consideration of cardiac causes of dizziness are also important. Useful basic screening tools are ECG and postural blood pressures, but a low threshold for prolonged cardiac monitoring, echocardiograpy, and cardiology opinion is advisable.

Depression/Anxiety

Depression and anxiety are very common following mild TBI. Two basic screening questions focussing on the two core symptoms of depression ('During the last month have you often been bothered by feeling down, depressed, or hopeless?' and 'Do you have little interest or pleasure in doing things?') have excellent sensitivity, albeit modest specificity, and are a useful way of establishing if more detailed evaluation is required (17). The DSM-5 criteria for depression and anxiety are outlined in Table 4 (18). Risk assessment for deliberate self-harm and suicide are vital components and urgent specialist

Table 4 DSM-5 diagnostic criteria for depression and anxiety (18)

DSM-5 criteria for a major depressive episode	DSM-5 features of generalised anxiety disorder

• An individual must be experiencing five or more symptoms of depression during the same two-week period and at least one of the symptoms should be either (1) depressed mood or (2) loss of interest or pleasure
• Symptoms of depression:
  o Depressed mood
  o Markedly diminished interest or pleasure in most or all activities
  o Significant weight loss (or poor appetite) or weight gain
  o Insomnia or hypersomnia
  o Psychomotor retardation
  o Fatigue or loss of energy
  o Feelings of worthlessness or excessive or inappropriate guilt
  o Diminished ability to think or concentrate, or indecisiveness
  o Recurrent thoughts of death (not just fear of dying), or suicidal ideation, plan, or attempt
  o Sleep disturbance
	• Excessive anxiety and worry (apprehensive expectation), occurring more days than not for at least six months, about a number of events or activities (such as work or school performance)
	• The individual finds it difficult to control the worry
	• Anxiety and worry are associated with three (or more) of the following six symptoms (with at least some symptoms present for more days than not for the past six months): restlessness or feeling 'keyed up' or on edge, easily fatigued, difficulty concentrating or mind going blank, irritability, muscle tension, sleep disturbance (difficulty falling or staying asleep, or restless, unsatisfying sleep)
	• The anxiety, worry, or physical symptoms cause clinically significant distress or impairment in social, occupational, or other important areas of functioning
	• The disturbance is not attributable to the psychological effects of a substance, and cannot be explained by another mental disorder

input is required if a patient is felt to be at high risk. It should be noted that although sleep disturbance and fatigue are commonly associated with depression, they can occur independently from affective symptoms in the context of TBI and have been shown to be related to impaired endogenous melatonin production and low dose melatonin can be helpful (19).

There is good evidence for targeted psychological interventions such as cognitive behavioural therapy for both anxiety and depression (20). In terms of medications, selective serotonin inhibitors such as escitalopram and sertraline are often favoured owing to their efficacy, limited side effect profile, and interactions with other medications, but agents with broader mechanism of action such as tri-cyclic antidepressants may be helpful in the context of co-morbid migraine (21).

In addition to depression and anxiety, it is becoming increasingly recognised that there is also an increased risk of post-traumatic stress disorder following a mild TBI, particularly if the injury results from assault or other violence (22). Specialist psychiatry and psychology input is of great value in this setting.

Functional Neurological Symptoms

It is becoming increasingly recognised that functional neurological symptoms are more common in the context of mild TBI (23). The core clinical feature of functional neurological symptoms is 'internal inconsistency', a prime example being Hoover's sign in the context of leg weakness (i.e. weakness of voluntary hip extension with normal involuntary hip extension during contralateral hip flexion against resistance) (24). A positive diagnosis and explanation of functional neurological symptoms is a key step of management. Patient education resources such as neurosymptoms.org can be helpful in this regard. Cognitive behavioural therapy, physiotherapy, and assessment by specialist multidisciplinary clinics with expertise in functional neurological disorders are the mainstays of ongoing management.

Cognitive Symptoms

Cognitive symptoms are commonly reported by patients with mild TBI and can be difficult to disentangle. Neuropsychological input is particularly helpful as detailed testing can often identify impairments in specific cognitive domains, which can be interpreted in the context of pre-morbid estimates of function, educational background, as well as other factors such as low mood. This can often feed into therapeutic avenues such as psychoeducation, cognitive behavioural therapy, as well as informing practical considerations such as return to work. Charitable organisations such as Headway (www.headway.org.uk/) are also an invaluable resource for patients.

Importance of Neuropsychiatry and Neuropsychology

As highlighted in the previous section, there are a wide range of symptoms that may follow a mild TBI. Many of these symptoms are either psychiatric/psychological (e.g. anxiety/depression) or may have a significant psychological impact (e.g. disabling symptoms of a headache/dizziness). Furthermore, there are multiple biological, psychological, and social factors, some of which may be premorbid, that can influence outcome following head injury. The complex interplay between these factors, as well as the biological effects of head injury, likely account for a significant portion of heterogeneity seen in this patient population (23). Disentangling these aspects can pose a considerable challenge, and specialist input from neuropsychiatrists and clinical neuropsychologists with expertise in head injury is often vital in effectively managing patients with mild TBI.

Investigations in Mild TBI

Computed Tomography

Computed Tomography (CT) scans are the cornerstone of investigation in head injury. They have a wide range of benefits, including cost and availability. They are particularly useful in the context of head injury for diagnosing moderate–severe (definite) TBI and identifying patients who require urgent neurosurgical intervention. In the United Kingdom, there are specific guidelines around the use of CT head scans developed by the National Institute for Health and Care Excellence (NICE) (Table 5) (25). However, the vast majority of CT scans in the

Table 5 NICE guidelines for CT head in the emergency department (www.nice.org.uk/guidance/ng232)

NICE guidelines for CT head	Adults
Within 1 hour	• GCS <13 on initial assessment • GCS <15 at 2 hours after the injury on assessment • Suspected open or depressed skull fracture • Any sign of basal skull fracture (haemotympanum, 'panda' eyes, cerebrospinal fluid leakage from the ear or nose, Battle's sign) • Post-traumatic seizure • Focal neurological deficit • More than one episode of vomiting
Within 8 hours	• Age >65 years • Any history of bleeding or clotting disorders • Dangerous mechanism of injury (a pedestrian or cyclist struck by a motor vehicle, an occupant ejected from a motor vehicle, or a fall from a height of more than 1 metre or five stairs) • More than 30 minutes of retrograde amnesia of events immediately before the head injury

context of head injury are normal, which has the potential to create a false sense of reassurance to both the clinician and the patient.

Magnetic Resonance Imaging

As is the case with CT head imaging, standard MRI brain scans are often normal in mild TBI. However, there are specific advanced MRI techniques which are proving to be clinically useful in mild TBI.

T2*-weighted gradient-echo (GRE) and susceptibility weight imaging are sensitive to the paramagnetic effects of iron, which enables them to detect small foci of hypointensity known as microbleeds (Figure 2). Microbleeds are a biomarker of traumatic vascular injury and have been shown to be present in up to 27% of patients with mild TBI. They have also been a predictor of poor outcome (26).

In addition to traumatic vascular injury, traumatic axonal injury has been shown to be a key predictor of outcomes in TBI, but historically has been difficult to detect clinically. Advanced diffusion weight MRI techniques such as Diffusion Tensor Imaging (DTI) have the ability to estimate the microstructural integrity of cerebral white matter and have been proposed as a marker of traumatic axonal injury in vivo. A landmark study of veterans from the Iraq and Afghanistan wars revealed evidence of DTI abnormalities in 29% of soldiers with a diagnosis of mild TBI from a blast injury and normal conventional brain imaging (27). Research in this area has progressed and validated pipelines exist that allow DTI to be applied to individual patients to detect individuals with and without DTI abnormalities (Figure 3). This is being applied clinically in some centres and is likely to be a useful tool going forward in assessing patients with mild TBI (28).

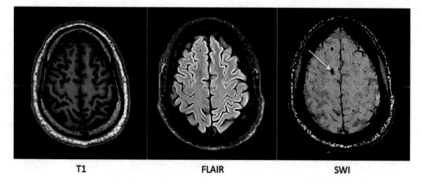

Figure 2 Example of a microbleed visible on blood sensitive sequence (5). Reproduced under Creative Commons Attribution licence.

Case study 1

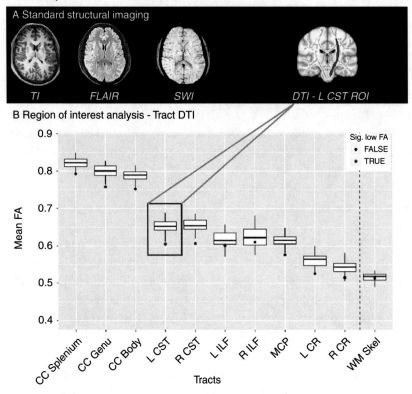

Figure 3 Example of DTI abnormalities in an individual with a history
of mild TBI in the context of professional rugby. Standard MRI
sequences in panel A demonstrated no abnormalities. Panel B demonstrates an
individual analysis of mean FA (fractional anisotropy) in selected
tracts of interest. Box plots show the normal range in healthy age-matched
controls. Black dots represent where a value is not abnormal, while
red points indicate where an individual has a significantly abnormal FA
compared to the control cohort. In this case there is evidence of abnormal FA in
the genu of the corpus callosum (CC Genu), as well as left and right
corticospinal tracts (L CST and R CST) suggestive of traumatic
axonal injury (29). Reproduced under Creative Commons
Attribution licence.

Blood-Based Biomarkers

Although not in routine clinical practice, research into blood-based biomarkers
of mild TBI is rapidly expanding. Plasma neurofilament light levels, a marker of
axonal injury, and plasma glial fibrillary acidic protein, a biomarker of astrocyte

activation and neuroinflammation, are key examples that are both elevated post mild TBI and have been shown to predict symptom duration and abnormalities on imaging (30,31).

Pitfalls and Pearls in Mild TBI

- Avoid broad terms such as 'post-concussive' syndrome and focus on individual symptoms and develop a tailored investigation and management plan
- Loss of consciousness and post-traumatic amnesia can be difficult to diagnose in retrospect and collateral information is crucial
- Migraine is a very common but treatable cause of morbidity in mild TBI
- Avoid opioids in mild TBI
- Always perform positional testing to look for BPPV for patients presenting with dizziness post head injury and have a low threshold for involving specialists (i.e. audiovestibular medicine/neuro-otology)
- In patients presenting with acute onset persistent dizziness following trauma have a low threshold for imaging of neck vessels (CT/MR angiogram) and MRI brain to exclude posterior circulation stroke secondary to vertebral artery dissection
- Always screen for depression in mild TBI
- Specialist neuropsychologists/neuropsychiatric input is invaluable
- CT head is often normal in mild TBI, but should not be considered as reassuring
- Blood-sensitive and diffusion-weighted MRI sequences are useful for identifying evidence of traumatic vascular and traumatic axonal injury, respectively.

Guidelines

Head injury: assessment and early management. NICE guideline published 18 May 2023. www.nice.org.uk/guidance/ng232.

References

1. National Clinical Guideline Centre (UK). *Head Injury: Triage, Assessment, Investigation and Early Management of Head Injury in Children, Young People and Adults [Internet]*. London: National Institute for Health and Care Excellence (UK); 2014 [cited 15 May 2022]. (National Institute for Health and Clinical Excellence: Guidance). www.ncbi.nlm.nih.gov/books/ NBK248061/.
2. Lawrence T, Helmy A, Bouamra O, et al. Traumatic brain injury in England and Wales: Prospective audit of epidemiology, complications and standardised mortality. BMJ Open. 24 November 2016;6(11):e012197.
3. Carroll LJ, Cassidy JD, Holm L, Kraus J, Coronado VG, WHO Collaborating Centre Task Force on Mild Traumatic Brain Injury. Methodological issues and research recommendations for mild traumatic brain injury: The WHO Collaborating Centre Task force on mild traumatic brain injury. J Rehabil Med. February 2004;(43 Suppl):113–25.
4. Malec JF, Brown AW, Leibson CL, et al. The Mayo classification system for traumatic brain injury severity. J Neurotrauma. September 2007;24 (9):1417–24.
5. Sharp DJ, Jenkins PO. Concussion is confusing us all. Pract Neurol. June 2015;15(3):172–86.
6. Yuh EL, Jain S, Sun X, et al. Pathological computed tomography features associated with adverse outcomes after mild traumatic brain injury: A TRACK-TBI study with external validation in CENTER-TBI. JAMA Neurol. 1 September 2021;78(9):1137–48.
7. Hou R, Moss-Morris R, Peveler R, et al. When a minor head injury results in enduring symptoms: A prospective investigation of risk factors for post-concussional syndrome after mild traumatic brain injury. J Neurol Neurosurg Psychiatry. February 2012;83(2):217–23.
8. Papa L, Mendes ME, Braga CF. Mild traumatic brain injury among the geriatric population. Curr Transl Geriatr Exp Gerontol Rep. 1 September 2012;1(3):135–42.
9. Parker TD, Rees R, Rajagopal S, et al. Post-traumatic amnesia. Pract Neurol. April 2022;22(2):129–37.
10. Nakase-Richardson R, Sherer M, Seel RT, et al. Utility of post-traumatic amnesia in predicting 1-year productivity following traumatic brain injury: Comparison of the Russell and Mississippi PTA classification intervals. J Neurol Neurosurg Psychiatry. May 2011;82(5):494–9.

11. Ponsford J, Janzen S, McIntyre A, et al. INCOG recommendations for management of cognition following traumatic brain injury, part I: Posttraumatic amnesia/delirium. J Head Trauma Rehabil. August 2014;29 (4):307–20.

12. Lucas S, Hoffman JM, Bell KR, Dikmen S. A prospective study of prevalence and characterization of headache following mild traumatic brain injury. Cephalalgia. February 2014;34(2):93–102.

13. Headache Classification Committee of the International Headache Society (IHS). The international classification of headache disorders, 3rd ed. (beta version). Cephalalgia. July 2013;33(9):629–808.

14. Sinclair AJ, Sturrock A, Davies B, Matharu M. Headache management: Pharmacological approaches. Pract Neurol. December 2015;15(6):411–23.

15. Smith RM, Marroney N, Beattie J, et al. A mixed methods randomised feasibility trial investigating the management of benign paroxysmal positional vertigo in acute traumatic brain injury. Pilot Feasibility Stud. 2020;6:130.

16. Kaski D, Bronstein AM. Epley and beyond: An update on treating positional vertigo. Pract Neurol. August 2014;14(4):210–21.

17. Bosanquet K, Bailey D, Gilbody S, et al. Diagnostic accuracy of the Whooley questions for the identification of depression: A diagnostic meta-analysis. BMJ Open. 9 December 2015;5(12):e008913.

18. Regier DA, Kuhl EA, Kupfer DJ. The DSM-5: Classification and criteria changes. World Psychiatry. June 2013;12(2):92–8.

19. Shekleton JA, Parcell DL, Redman JR, et al. Sleep disturbance and melatonin levels following traumatic brain injury. Neurology. 25 May 2010;74 (21):1732–8.

20. Waldron B, Casserly LM, O'Sullivan C. Cognitive behavioural therapy for depression and anxiety in adults with acquired brain injury: What works for whom? Neuropsychol Rehabil. 2013;23(1):64–101.

21. Cipriani A, Furukawa TA, Salanti G, et al. Comparative efficacy and acceptability of 21 antidepressant drugs for the acute treatment of adults with major depressive disorder: A systematic review and network meta-analysis. Lancet. 7 April 2018;391(10128):1357–66.

22. Stein MB, Jain S, Giacino JT, et al. Risk of posttraumatic stress disorder and major depression in civilian patients after mild traumatic brain injury: A TRACK-TBI study. JAMA Psychiatry. 1 March 2019;76(3):249–58.

23. Clark CN, Edwards MJ, Ong BE, et al. Reframing postconcussional syndrome as an interface disorder of neurology, psychiatry and psychology. Brain. 30 June 2022;145(6):1906–15.

24. Stone J, Zeman A, Sharpe M. Functional weakness and sensory disturbance. J Neurol Neurosurg Psychiatry. September 2002;73(3):241–5.

25. Rajesh S, Wonderling D, Bernstein I, Balson C, Lecky F, Guideline Committee. Head injury: Assessment and early management-summary of updated NICE guidance. BMJ. 30 May 2023;381:1130.

26. Griffin AD, Turtzo LC, Parikh GY, et al. Traumatic microbleeds suggest vascular injury and predict disability in traumatic brain injury. Brain. 1 November 2019;142(11):3550–64.

27. MacDonald CL, Johnson AM, Cooper D, et al. Detection of blast-related traumatic brain injury in U.S. military personnel. N Engl J Med. 2 June 2011;364(22):2091–100.

28. Jolly AE, Bălăeţ M, Azor A, et al. Detecting axonal injury in individual patients after traumatic brain injury. Brain. 12 February 2021;144(1):92–113.

29. Zimmerman KA, Laverse E, Samra R, et al. White matter abnormalities in active elite adult rugby players. Brain Communications. 1 July 2021;3(3): fcab133.

30. Shahim P, Zetterberg H, Tegner Y, Blennow K. Serum neurofilament light as a biomarker for mild traumatic brain injury in contact sports. Neurology. 9 May 2017;88(19):1788–94.

31. Bazarian JJ, Biberthaler P, Welch RD, et al. Serum GFAP and UCH-L1 for prediction of absence of intracranial injuries on head CT (ALERT-TBI): A multicentre observational study. Lancet Neurol. September 2018;17 (9):782–9.

Cambridge Elements ≡

Emergency Neurosurgery

Nihal Gurusinghe
Lancashire Teaching Hospital NHS Trust

Professor Nihal Gurusinghe is a Consultant Neurosurgeon at the Lancashire Teaching Hospitals NHS Trust. He is on the Executive Council of the Society of British Neurological Surgeons as the Lead for NICE (National Institute for Health and Care Excellence) guidelines relating to neurosurgical practice. He is also an examiner for the UK and International FRCS examinations in Neurosurgery.

Peter Hutchinson
University of Cambridge, Society of British Neurological Surgeons and Royal College of Surgeons of England

Peter Hutchinson BSc MBBS FFSEM FRCS(SN) PhD FMedSci is Professor of Neurosurgery and Head of the Division of Academic Neurosurgery at the University of Cambridge, and Honorary Consultant Neurosurgeon at Addenbrooke's Hospital. He is Director of Clinical Research at the Royal College of Surgeons of England and Meetings Secretary of the Society of British Neurological Surgeons.

Ioannis Fouyas
Royal College of Surgeons of Edinburgh

Ioannis Fouyas is a Consultant Neurosurgeon in Edinburgh. His clinical interests focus on the treatment of complex cerebrovascular and skull base pathologies. His academic endeavours concentrate in the field of cerebrovascular pathophysiology. His passion is technical surgical training, fulfilled in collaboration with the Royal College of Surgeons of Edinburgh. Finally, he pursues Undergraduate Neuroscience teaching, with a particular focus on functional Neuroanatomy.

Naomi Slator
North Bristol NHS Trust

Naomi Slator FRCS (SN) is a Consultant Spinal Neurosurgeon based at North Bristol NHS Trust. She has a specialist interest in Complex Spine alongside Cranial and Spinal Trauma. She completed her neurosurgical training in Birmingham and a six-month Fellowship in CSF and Trauma (2019). She then went on to complete her Spinal Fellowship in Leeds (2020) before moving to the southwest to take up her consultant post.

Ian Kamaly-Asl
Royal Manchester Children's Hospital

Ian Kamaly-Asl is a full time paediatric neurosurgeon and Honorary Chair at Royal Manchester Children's Hospital. He trained in North Western Deanery with fellowships at Boston Children's Hospital and Sick Kids in Toronto. Ian is a member of council of The Royal College of Surgeons of England and The SBNS where he is lead for mentoring and tackling oppressive behaviours.

Peter Whitfield

University Hospitals Plymouth NHS Trust

Professor Peter Whitfield is a Consultant Neurosurgeon at the South West Neurosurgical Centre, University Hospitals Plymouth NHS Trust. His clinical interests include vascular neurosurgery, neuro oncology and trauma. He has held many roles in postgraduate neurosurgical education and is President of the Society of British Neurological Surgeons. Peter has published widely, and is passionate about education, training and the promotion of clinical research.

About the Series

Elements in Emergency Neurosurgery is intended for trainees and practitioners in Neurosurgery and Emergency Medicine as well as allied specialties all over the world. Authored by international experts, this series provides core knowledge, common clinical pathways and recommendations on the management of acute conditions of the brain and spine.

Cambridge Elements ☰

Emergency Neurosurgery

Printed in the United States
by Baker & Taylor Publisher Services